WHEAT FREE DIET FOR BEGINNERS

Lose Weight Quickly, Achieve Optimal Health and Feel Energized with Gluten Free Recipes for Celiac Disease, Gluten Sensitivities, and Paleo Free Diets

EMMA ROSE

Table of Contents

Introduction

I want to thank you and congratulate you for purchasing this book!

This book contains proven steps and strategies on how to lose weight quickly and healthily with the Wheat Free Diet.

In this book, you will learn the basic principle of Wheat Free Diet and how you can use it to lose the pounds quickly without endangering your health. This eBook also contains easy and delicious recipes that you can use to begin your Wheat Free Diet.

Thanks again for purchasing this book, I hope you enjoy it! Please take some time to stop by and LIKE our Facebook page:

https://www.facebook.com/joypublishing

With gratitude,

Emma Rose

Chapter 1: About Wheat Free Diet

Is Wheat Bad for your Health?

According to William R. Davis, an American cardiologist and author of the book Wheat Belly, it is not the wheat that is the cause of his concern but the genetic changes that this plant underwent throughout the years. These genetic changes cause a person to gain weight or acquire allergies when consuming wheat.

What is Wheat Belly and Wheat Free Diet?

Wheat belly is the acquired fat found in the abdomen caused by consuming wheat. What Dr. Davis calls as wheat belly is often termed as "muffin top" bellies or "love handles". Severe wheat belly cases often looks like a stomach of a near-term pregnancy.

Meanwhile, Wheat Free Diet prohibits consumption of any forms of wheat. Most people who have undergone this diet have lost almost a pound per day during the first 10 days of dieting. And all of that without limiting calorie consumption, cutting fats, or imposing strict portion sizes.

Complete elimination of wheat results to lesser cravings, less hunger, and healthier food. By removing wheat, you have removed the main cause of fat accumulation in the abdomen area.

Wheat is an ingredient that is in nearly every food. How can you completely remove wheat from a person's diet?

There are many wheat alternatives that you can use. In the following chapters, you'll discover how you can still make wheat products without the wheat.

What Foods are Okay to Eat?

Real and natural foods like fruits, vegetables, and organic products. The only thing that you have to keep in mind is to stay away from wheat and overly processed products. Practice reading labels and avoid foods which contain hard-to-pronounce ingredients (in other words, you have to stay away from synthetically-made ingredients, such as preservatives and anticaking agents).

Chapter 2: Recipes for Breakfast

Dairy Free Pancakes

Ingredients:

- 1 ½ cups of finely ground blanched almond flour
- ½ tsp of baking soda
- ¼ tsp of salt
- ½ tsp of cinnamon
- 3 pcs of large eggs
- 5 tbsp of full fat coconut milk
- 2 tbsp of honey
- 1 tsp of vanilla
- ¼ cup of strawberries
- Oil, for cooking

Procedure:

1. Prepare a large mixing bowl. Sift the almond flour, baking soda, salt, and cinnamon into the bowl and stir to combine.

2. In a separate mixing bowl, add in the eggs, coconut milk, honey, and vanilla. Whisk the ingredients together until properly incorporated. Pour the mixture into the mixing bowl with the flour mixture. Stir the ingredients until they form a smooth batter. Then, set the mixture aside.

3. Prepare a skillet and heat the oil. Don't let the pan get too hot or the pancakes will stick.

4. Pour the batter into the pan and lower the heat if necessary. Flip the pancake once the edges are just starting

to form and the topside is bubbly. Fry until the pancake is cooked through.

5. Top with honey or maple syrup and sliced fruits.

Breakfast Bars

Ingredients:

- 1 ¼ cup of almond flour (pick the blanched variant)
- ¼ tsp of bay salt (rock salt should be fine)
- ¼ tsp of baking soda
- ¼ cup of grape seed oil
- ¼ cup of agave nectar
- 1 tsp of vanilla extract
- ½ cup of unsweetened shredded coconut
- ½ cup of pumpkin seeds
- ½ cup of sunflower seeds
- ¼ cup of blanched slivered almonds
- ¼ cup of raisins

Procedure:

1. In a small mixing bowl, combine the almond flour, baking soda, and Celtic sea salt. Stir the ingredients together.

2. In a large mixing bowl, combine the grape seed oil, vanilla extract, and agave nectar. Stir until the ingredients are well mixed. Gradually add in the almond flour mixture into the bowl and mix well.

3. Add in the shredded coconut, pumpkin seeds, almond slivers, sunflower seeds, and raisins. Stir the ingredients together until well incorporated.

4. Prepare an 8" x 8" baking dish and slightly grease it using the grape seed oil. Place the dough on the baking dish. Spread it evenly and pat it down using a spatula or with your bare hands.

5. Place the baking dish inside the oven and bake for 20 minutes at 350°F. Once cooking time is done, place the bars on a cooling pan and let them cool for two hours before serving.

Matzo Ball Soup

Ingredients:

- 4 pcs of eggs
- 2 tsp of Celtic sea salt
- ¼ tsp of pepper
- 2 cups of blanched almond flour, already sifted
- 6 cups of chicken or vegetable stock

Procedure:

1. In a mixing bowl, add in the eggs, pepper, and 1 teaspoon of salt. Beat the ingredients together for 2 minutes. Add in the almond flour and stir. Place the bowl inside the refrigerator and wait for 4 hours.

2. Place a large pot on a stove and fill it with water. Add in the remaining teaspoon of sea salt and bring the water to a boil.

3. Remove the mixture from the refrigerator. Wash your hands and take the refrigerated batter and roll it into 1" balls, then add them into the boiling water. Do the same with the remaining batter. Reduce the heat and place a lid over the pot and let it simmer for about 20 minutes.

4. In a separate pot, heat the chicken or vegetable stock.

5. When the matzo balls are finished cooking, remove it from the simmering water and place it into the pot with the chicken or vegetable stock.

Silver Dollar Pancakes

Ingredients:

- 3 pcs of large eggs
- 1 tbsp of water
- 1 tbsp of vanilla extract
- 2 tbsp of agave nectar
- 1 ½ cups of blanched almond flour
- ¼ tsp of Celtic sea salt
- ¼ tsp of baking soda

Procedure:

1. In a large mixing bowl, combine the eggs, vanilla extract, water, and agave nectar. Whisk the ingredients together until properly incorporated.

2. Add in the almond flour, baking soda, and Celtic sea salt. Stir until the ingredients form a smooth batter.

3. Prepare a skillet and heat coconut or grape seed oil over medium heat.

4. Use a large tablespoon to scoop the batter on the skillet. Cook the pancakes one at a time. When the batter becomes bubbly, flip the pancakes to cook the other side. Repeat the procedure with the rest of the batter.

Cinnamon Buns

Ingredients:

<u>*for the toppings:*</u>
- 2 tbsp of agave nectar
- 1 tbsp of ground cinnamon
- 1 tbsp of grape seed oil

<u>*for the bun:*</u>
- 1 cup of blanched almond flour
- 2 tbsp of coconut flour
- ½ tsp of baking soda
- ¼ tsp of Celtic sea salt
- ¼ cup of grape seed oil
- ¼ cup of agave nectar
- 3 pcs of eggs
- 1 tbsp of vanilla extract

Procedure:

1. Make the toppings by combining the agave nectar, ground cinnamon, and grape seed oil. Whisk the ingredients together until well-mixed. Then, set it aside.

2. In a large mixing bowl, combine the almond flour, baking soda, coconut flour, and salt. Stir the ingredients together.

3. Add in the agave nectar, grape seed oil, eggs, and vanilla extract. Whisk the ingredients together until it forms a smooth batter.

4. Prepare a muffin tin and line it with muffin cups. Scoop the batter into the muffin cups filling about ¼ of the way. Then, add in the toppings. Do the same with the rest of the batter and toppings.

5. Place the muffin tin inside the oven and bake for 8 to 12 minutes at 350F. Once done baking, let it cool for two hours. Best enjoyed with cream cheese frosting.

Chapter 3: Recipes for Bread and Muffins

Pumpkin and Walnut Muffins

Ingredients:

- 1 cup of almond flour
- 1 cup of canned pumpkin
- 2 pcs of eggs
- ¼ cup of almond butter
- ¼ cup of honey
- 1 tsp of baking powder
- 1 tsp of cinnamon
- ½ tsp of pumpkin pie spice
- ¼ tsp of salt
- ¾ cup of chopped walnuts

Procedure:

1. Turn on the oven and set it to 350°F.

2. In a large mixing bowl, combine the almond flour, pumpkin, eggs, almond butter, honey, baking powder, cinnamon, pumpkin pie spice, salt, and walnuts. Stir the ingredients until well mixed.

3. Prepare a muffin tin and lightly grease it with cooking spray or use muffin liners. Divide the batter into six equal cups of muffin and pour it into the muffin tin.

4. Place the muffin tin inside the oven and bake for 32 to 35 minutes. Once cooked, place the muffins on a wire rack to let them cool before serving.

Blueberry Muffins

Ingredients:

- 1 cup of almond butter
- 1 cup of almond flour
- 3 pcs of eggs, already whisked
- ½ cup of raw honey
- 1/3 cup of shredded coconut
- 1/3 cup of coconut oil, already melted
- ½ tsp of baking soda
- ½ tsp of baking powder
- ¼ tsp of sea salt
- A pinch of cinnamon
- ½ cup of fresh blueberries

Procedure:

1. Turn on the oven and set it to 350°F.

2. In a large mixing bowl, add in the almond butter, almond flour, whisked eggs, raw honey, shredded coconut, virgin coconut oil, baking soda, baking powder, sea salt, cinnamon, and blueberries. Stir the ingredients together until well mixed.

3. Prepare a muffin tin and line it with paper liners. Divide the batter into 8 to 10 muffin cups and pour it in the muffin tin.

4. Place the muffin tin inside the oven and bake for 15 to 20 minutes. Let the muffins cool before serving.

Peach Coconut Muffins

Ingredients:

- 1 ½ cups of almond flour
- ¼ cup of coconut flour
- ¼ cup of unsweetened shredded coconut flakes
- 1 tsp of cinnamon
- ½ tsp of baking soda
- ¼ tsp of salt
- 2 pcs of eggs
- ¼ cup of melted coconut oil
- Half of a banana, already mashed
- ¼ cup of unsweetened applesauce
- ½ tsp of vanilla extract
- 2/3 cup of peeled and diced peaches

Procedure:

1. Turn on the oven and set it to 350°F.

2. Prepare a muffin tin and lightly grease it with cooking oil or line it with muffin cups.

3. In a large mixing bowl, combine the almond and coconut flour, coconut flakes, ground cinnamon, baking soda, salt, eggs, coconut oil, mashed banana, applesauce, vanilla extract, and peaches. Stir the ingredients together until they form a smooth batter.

4. Pour the batter into the muffin tin, filling the cups about ¾ of the way. You can top each muffin with extra diced peaches if you like.

5. Place the muffin tin inside the oven and bake for 25 minutes. Once cooked, transfer the muffins into a cooling rack to cool completely.

Irish Soda Bread

Ingredients:

- 2 ¾ cups of blanched almond flour
- ¼ tsp of Celtic sea salt
- 1 ½ tsp of baking soda
- ½ cup of raisins
- 2 pcs of eggs
- 2 tbsp of agave nectar
- 2 tbsp of apple cider vinegar
- A pinch of caraway seeds

Procedure:

1. In a large mixing bowl, add in the almond flour, baking soda, Celtic sea salt, and raisins. Stir the ingredients to combine.

2. Add in the eggs, apple cider vinegar, and agave nectar into the bowl. Mix the ingredients together until properly combined.

3. Place the dough over a piece of parchment paper. Use a rolling pin to form the dough into an 8-in circle that is 1 ½-in thick.

4. Score the top of the dough about ½-in deep in the shape of a cross using a serrated knife. Sprinkle the caraway seeds evenly on the top of the dough.

5. Prepare a baking sheet and place the dough with the parchment paper on it. Place the baking sheet in the oven and bake for 20 minutes at 350°F. Once baking time has elapsed, turn off the oven and leave the bread inside for 10 minutes more.

6. Remove the baking sheet in the oven and let it cool for another 30 minutes before slicing and serving.

Chocolate Zucchini Bread

Ingredients:

- 1 ¼ cups of blanched almond flour
- ¼ cup of cacao powder
- ¼ tsp of Celtic sea salt
- ½ tsp of baking soda
- 2 pcs of large eggs
- 2 tbsp of coconut oil
- ¼ cup of honey
- ¼ tsp of vanilla stevia
- ¾ cup of zucchini, already grated

Procedure:

1. Add the cacao powder and almond flour in a large mixing bowl fit for a food processor. Mix the ingredients together.

2. Add in the Celtic sea salt and baking soda into the bowl and stir again.

3. Add in the eggs, honey, coconut oil, vanilla stevia, and zucchini. Use the food processor to mix the ingredients. Blend until the ingredients are well-incorporated.

4. Prepare a 6.5" x 4" loaf pan. Lightly grease the pan using coconut oil and dust it with almond flour. Pour the batter inside the loaf pan and place it inside the oven.

5. Bake for 35 to 40 minutes at 350°F. Once done, let it cool on a wire rack for 2 hours.

Chapter 4: Recipes for Cakes and Cookies

Double Chocolate Chunk Cookies

Ingredients:

- 8 oz of bittersweet chocolate, melt the first half and coarsely chop the second half
- 1 ½ cups of almond flour
- ½ cup of unsweetened natural cocoa
- ½ tsp of baking soda
- ½ tsp of sea salt
- 1 stick of butter, sliced into cubes
- 1 cup of coconut sugar
- 2 pcs of large eggs
- 1 tsp of pure vanilla extract

Procedure:

1. Turn on the oven and set it to 350°F.

2. In a large mixing bowl, combine the unsweetened cocoa, almond flour, salt, baking soda, and sugar. Use a hand mixer or whisk to mix the ingredients.

3. Add in the cubes of butter and process until they're combined with the dry ingredients. Then, add in the eggs, vanilla extract, and melted chocolate into the bowl. Blend the ingredients together until they becomes smooth. Stir in the chopped pieces of chocolate.

4. Prepare a baking sheet and line it with parchment paper. Drop a tablespoon of cookie mixture into the baking sheet and place each drop a few inches apart.

5. Place the baking sheets inside the oven and bake for 8 to 10 minutes. Rotate the baking sheets about halfway through the baking time. Bake the cookies until it has just set. Then, transfer the cookies into a wire rack and let it cool completely.

Banana Cake

Ingredients:

- 3 cups of blanched almond flour
- ½ tsp of Celtic sea salt
- 1 tsp of baking soda
- ¼ cup of agave nectar
- ¼ cup of grape seed oil
- 3 pcs of eggs, already whisked
- 1 tbsp of vanilla extract
- 2 pcs of bananas, already mashed

Procedure:

1. In a large mixing bowl, combine the almond flour, baking soda, and Celtic sea salt. Stir the ingredients together.

2. In another bowl, add in the agave nectar, whisked eggs, grape seed oil, mashed bananas, and vanilla extract. Mix until properly combined. Add this mixture into the large bowl with the almond flour mix. Stir until properly incorporated.

3. Prepare a 9" cake pan or two small loaf pans and pour the batter inside.

4. Place the pan inside the oven and bake for 40 minutes at 350°F. Once cooked, remove the cake from the oven and set it aside to cool.

Cabernet Cookies

Ingredients:

- 1 ¼ cups of almond flour (choose the blanched variant)
- ¼ tsp of sea salt (any kind should be fine)
- ¼ tsp of baking soda
- ¼ cup of grape seed oil
- ¼ cup of agave nectar
- ¼ cup of grape seed flour
- ¼ cup of chocolate chunks

Procedure:

1. In a large mixing bowl, add in the almond flour, sea salt, baking soda, and grape seed flour. Stir the ingredients together.

2. In a smaller bowl, combine the grape seed oil and agave nectar. Stir then pour the mixture into the bowl with the flour mixture. Mix until all the ingredients are properly incorporated.

3. Fold in the chocolate chunks until evenly distributed.

4. Prepare a baking sheet and line it with parchment paper. Use your hands or a spoon to form ½-in balls. Then press the dough into the baking sheet to form a cookie shape.

5. Place the baking sheet inside the oven and bake for 7 to 10 minutes at 350°F. Once cooked, let it cool completely before serving.

Black and White Cookies

Ingredients:

- 2 ½ cups of blanched almond flour
- ½ tsp of Celtic sea salt
- ¼ cup of agave nectar
- ½ cup of grape seed oil
- 1 tbsp of vanilla extract
- 1 cup of chocolate chunks

Procedure:

1. In a large mixing bowl, add in the almond flour and Celtic sea salt. Stir the ingredients together. Add in the agave nectar, grape seed oil, and vanilla extract. Mix the ingredients together until well incorporated.

2. Place the dough inside the freezer for about 30 minutes.

3. Prepare two pieces of parchment paper. Place the dough in between the pieces of papers and roll it out to about ¼-in thick.

4. Prepare a baking sheet and line it with parchment paper. Cut the cookie dough using a 2-in cookie cutter and place the cookies on the baking sheet.

5. Once the dough is all used up, place the baking sheet in the oven and bake for 5 to 7 minutes at 350°F. Place the cookies on a wire rack and let them cool for 30 minutes.

6. Prepare a small saucepan and add in the chocolate chunks. Place it over low heat and melt the chocolate while stirring continuously (make sure that nothing is beginning to stick to the bottom).

7. Once the chocolate is completely melted, remove the pan from the heat and get the cooled down cookies. Dip the cookies about halfway into the chocolate and place it on a baking sheet with parchment paper to let it cool. You can also place it inside the refrigerator if you like.

Carrot Cake

Ingredients:

- 3 cups of blanched almond flour
- 1 tsp of Celtic sea salt
- 1 tsp of baking soda
- 1 tbsp of ground cinnamon
- 1 tsp of nutmeg
- 5 pcs of eggs
- ½ cup of agave nectar
- ¼ cup of grapeseed oil
- 3 cups of carrots, already grated
- 1 cup of raisins
- 1 cup of walnuts

Procedure:

1. In a mixing bowl (big enough to prevent spillage), add in the flour, Celtic sea salt, baking soda, nutmeg, and ground cinnamon. Stir everything together until well combined.

2. In a separate mixing bowl, add in the eggs, grapeseed oil, and agave nectar. Whisk the ingredients together then add in the carrots, walnuts, and raisins. Stir the ingredients together then pour the mixture into the bowl that contains the almond flour mixture.

3. Mix the ingredients together until properly combined.

4. Prepare two 9" round cake pans and grease it lightly. Pour the batter into the pans and place it inside the oven. Bake for 35 minutes at 325°F.

5. Once baked, place it on a wire rack and let it cool. Spread with coconut cream frosting for better results.

Chocolate Strawberry Shortcake

Ingredients:

- 1 ½ cups of almond flour (the blanched variety works best)
- ¼ cup of coconut flour
- 2 tbsp of cacao powder
- ¼ tsp of Celtic sea salt
- ½ tsp of baking soda
- 3 pcs of eggs
- ½ cup of agave nectar

For the topping:
- 2 cups of heavy cream
- 2 tbsp of agave nectar
- 1 tbsp of vanilla extract
- 1 lb of fresh strawberries, already hulled and sliced

Procedure:

1. In a large mixing bowl, combine the almond flour, cacao powder, coconut flour, baking soda, and sea salt. Stir the ingredients together.

2. Add in the agave nectar and eggs. Mix the ingredients they're completely combined.

3. Prepare a baking sheet and line it with parchment paper. Using a tablespoon, scoop the batter into the baking sheet.

4. Place the baking sheet in the oven. Baking the biscuits for 12 to 15 minutes at 350°F should be enough. Once done baking, let the biscuits cool on a wire rack.

5. In a mixing bowl, combine the heavy cream, agave nectar, and vanilla extract. Whip the ingredients together until properly combined.

6. Once completely cooled, slice the biscuits in half, horizontally. Arrange the bottom halves on the baking sheet and place a dollop of cream and a slice of strawberry. Top with the remaining half of the biscuit and top with another dollop of cream and strawberry.

Chapter 5: Recipes for Snacks

Chocolate Pecan Bars

Ingredients:

- ½ cup of pecans
- 6 tbsp of coconut oil, already melted
- 1 tbsp of raw honey
- 1 cup of almond flour
- 5 tbsp of water
- 2 tbsp of coconut oil, already melted
- ¼ cup of raw cacao powder
- 2 tbsp of raw honey
- 1 tsp of vanilla extract
- 2 pcs of eggs
- A pinch of salt
- A handful of raw pecans

Ingredients:

1. Turn on the oven and set it to 350°F.

2. Prepare an 8" x 8" baking pan and line it with parchment paper. Make sure that all sides are covered.

3. In a food processor, add in ½ cup of pecans and process until it is coarsely ground. Pour the pecans in a large mixing bowl and add in the 6 tablespoons of coconut oil, 1 tablespoon of raw honey, and almond flour. Mix the ingredients until thoroughly combined.

4. Pour the mixture into the baking pan and spread it evenly across the bottom. Place the baking pan in the oven and bake for 12 minutes.

5. While baking, combine the water, cacao powder, 2 tablespoons of coconut oil, raw cacao powder, 2 tablespoons of raw honey, eggs, salt, and vanilla extract in a mixing bowl. Whisk the ingredients together until properly incorporated.

6. Remove the baking pan from the oven once cooking time is done and pour the mixture over the crust. Spread it evenly and return the baking pan in the oven. Bake for another 12 minutes or until the chocolate is set.

7. Chop the raw pecans and sprinkle it over the baked pecan bars. Let it cool completely before slicing and serving.

Pizza

Ingredients:

- 3 cups of almond flour
- 1/3 cup of coconut flour
- ¼ cup of unflavored whey protein powder
- 2 tsp of baking powder
- 2 tsp of garlic powder
- ¾ tsp of salt
- 4 pcs of eggs, beaten lightly
- ½ cup of butter, already melted
- ¼ cup of almond milk
- Your favorite pizza toppings

Procedure:

1. Turn on the oven and set it to 350°F.

2. In a large mixing bowl, combine the almond flour, coconut flour, baking powder, whey protein, salt, and garlic powder. Stir to combine the ingredients together.

3. Add in the eggs, butter, and almond milk and stir until all the ingredients are combined. The mixture will be slightly sticky.

4. Divide the dough in half and form each one into a ball. Place a parchment paper underneath and over the dough ball. Use a rolling pin to flatten the dough balls to form small discs about ½-in thick.

5. Remove the parchment paper on top of the dough and place the unbaked crust together with the bottom layer of parchment paper into a baking sheet.

6. Place the baking sheet in the oven and bake for 8 minutes. Remove the sheet from the oven and add in your favorite pizza toppings. Replace the baking sheet into the oven and bake for another 5 to 7 minutes.

7. Once the cheese has melted, remove the pizza from the oven and let it sit for 5 minutes to cool down slightly. Do the same with the remaining dough.

Strawberry Scones

Ingredients:

- 4 pcs of eggs, already beaten
- 3 cups of almond flour
- 3 tbsp of pure maple syrup
- 2 tbsp of applesauce
- 3 tsp of baking powder
- 3 tsp of vanilla extract
- 1 ½ cups of strawberries, thinly sliced
- 2 cups of confectioner's sugar
- 2 tbsp of heavy cream

Procedure:

1. Turn on the oven and set it to 375°F.

2. Prepare a baking sheet and line it with parchment paper.

3. In a large mixing bowl, combine the eggs, almond flour, pure maple syrup, applesauce, baking powder, and vanilla extract. Mix the ingredients thoroughly then fold in the strawberries.

4. Place the dough on the baking sheet and form a large equilateral triangle. Then, slice the dough into smaller triangles carefully to prevent the dough from breaking apart.

5. Place the baking sheet inside the oven and bake for 15 to 20 minutes. Once cooked, remove from the oven and let it cool for about 10 minutes before serving.

6. In a small bowl, combine the confectioner's sugar and heavy cream. Whisk to mix well. Then, drizzle the icing over the cooled scones.

Orange Dark Chocolate Chip Scones

Ingredients:

- 2 cups of blanched almond flour
- ¾ tsp of baking soda
- ½ cup of chocolate chunks
- 1 tbsp of orange zest
- 1 pc of egg
- 3 tbsp of agave nectar

Procedure:

1. In a large mixing bowl, combine the almond flour, baking soda, orange zest, and chunks of chocolate. Stir until the ingredients are well-incorporated.

2. In a small bowl, combine the egg and agave nectar. Whisk the ingredients together until properly combined. Pour the contents over the flour mixture and stir until the ingredients are evenly distributed. You can use your hands to knead the dough.

3. Form the dough into a ½-in thick circle and slice it into eight equal pieces just like you would a pizza.

4. Prepare a baking sheet and line it with parchment paper. Place the scones on the baking sheet using a metal spatula to prevent them from breaking apart.

5. Turn on the oven and set it to 350°F.

6. Place the baking sheet inside the oven and bake for 10 to 15 minutes.

Goji Power Bars

Ingredients:

- 1 cup of blanched almond flour
- 1 tbsp of coconut flour
- 2 tbsp of golden flax meal
- ¼ tsp of Celtic sea salt
- ½ tsp of baking soda
- 2 tbsp of coconut sugar
- ¼ tsp of stevia
- 2 pcs of eggs
- ½ cup of goji berries, place the berries in ¼ cup of boiling water
- ½ cup of chocolate chunks

Procedure:

1. In a large mixing bowl, combine the almond flour, golden flax meal, coconut flour, baking soda, and Celtic sea salt. Stir the ingredients.

2. Add in the coconut sugar, eggs, and stevia into the bowl. Use a hand mixer to blend the ingredients together. Mix the ingredients until well-incorporated.

3. Add in the goji berries and chocolate chunks and stir. Make sure that the berries and chocolate are evenly distributed.

4. Prepare an 8" x 8" baking dish and pour the mixture inside. Use a spoon or spatula to spread the mixture across the bottom of the dish. Compress the mixture to make it about an inch thick.

5. Place the baking dish in the oven and bake for 15 minutes at 350°F. Once baked, let it cool before cutting it into small squares and serving.

Nacho Cheese Triangles

Ingredients:

- 2 cups of blanched almond flour
- 1 tsp of Celtic sea salt
- 1 tsp of baking soda
- 1 tsp of chipotle powder
- 1 tsp of chili powder
- 1 (8 oz) bar of cheddar cheese, grated
- 1 pc of large egg

Procedure:

1. In a large mixing bowl, add in the almond flour, baking soda, sea salt, chipotle powder, chili powder, and cheddar cheese. Stir the ingredients together.

2. In a small dish, whisk the eggs and add it into the mixing bowl.

3. Stir all the ingredients together until properly incorporated. You can use your hands to knead the dough to make sure that the ingredients are well-mixed.

4. Form the dough into a circle about half an inch thick. Slice it into 16 slices like you would a pizza.

5. Prepare a baking sheet and line it with parchment paper. Using a spatula, transfer the triangular dough into the baking sheet. Place the sheet into the oven and bake for 9 to 10 minutes at 375°F. This snack is best served with an avocado dip.

Conclusion

Thank you again for purchasing this book!

I hope this book was able to help you to learn about the wheat belly dilemma and the Wheat Free Diet. You now know how important it is to stay away from modern wheat, and you also know that doing that isn't really difficult.

The next step is to use this book to help ease your way into the diet and enjoy a healthier food lifestyle.

In addition, please remember to LIKE our Facebook page in order to find other resources and upcoming promotions:

https://www.facebook.com/joypublishing

With sincere thanks,

Emma Rose

Preview of 'Raw Food Diet Guide'
Lose Weight Quickly, Achieve Optimal Health and Feel Energized with the Raw Food Diet and Raw Food Recipes

Chapter 1
An Overview of the Raw Food Diet

The concept of the raw food diet is simple – cooking diminishes the nutritional value of food. Even though most of the food items in the diet are consumed while it is raw, heating is acceptable provided that the temperature stays between the range of 104 to 118°F or below.

Since cooking is perceived to kill off enzymes naturally found in food, raw food practitioners choose to avoid cooked food. As a matter of fact, overconsumption of cooked food forces the body to work overtime in order to produce more enzymes to support normal bodily functions. In the long run, the lack of enzymes can instigate a lot of problems involving a person's health, particularly accelerated aging, nutrient deficiency, weight gain and digestive problems.

Going raw can prove to be challenging, especially for those that are just starting out. It takes a lot of discipline to stick to the principles of the diet. Moreover, extra effort is required mentally and physically. When it comes to preparing your daily raw meals, your options are limited. Here are some of the procedures you may apply when organizing your meal plan:

- *Germination* – this is the process of soaking in water for a certain period of time. The recommended amount of time differs from one person to another but for raw foodists, the safest bet is to soak overnight.

- *Sprouting* – this comes after germination. After the beans, legumes or seeds are soaked, they may then be sprouted. Items should be left at room temperature until a sprout comes out of it. These sprouts may then be used for preparing food but should be rinsed and drained thoroughly beforehand.

- *Blending* – involves the use of a blender or food processor in order to create sauces, smoothies, or soup among others.

- *Dehydrating* – employs an equipment known as a dehydrator, which simulates sun drying. Common products of dehydrators are crackers, croutons, raisins, fruit leathers, sundried tomatoes, breads and kale chips.

- *Pickling* – a method of preserving food by marinating in a brine.

- *Juicing* – the process of extracting of vitamins, minerals and natural juices from plant tissues, particularly raw fruits and vegetables.

- *Fermentation* – process of converting sugar to carbon dioxide through the use of yeast.

Now that you know what procedures are available to you when preparing your raw meals, the next thing to know is which particular equipment/s you need to use. Below are some of the staple equipment that can be seen in every raw foodist's kitchen:

- *Dehydrator* – it is an enclosed container that has heating elements that can warm at low temperatures. It has a fan that blows warm air onto the food.

- *Spiral Slicer* – slices vegetables into spiral shapes

- *Thermometer* – to ensure that temperature stays below 118°F when heating food.

- *Trays* – for soaking and sprouting beans, legumes or seeds

- *Sprouters* or *mason jars*

These are the basic things you have to know if you intend to convert to the raw food diet. Now that you have an idea of what it is and how it works, you will then have to figure out why you would want to choose this lifestyle.

Check out the rest of this book on Amazon.

Or go to: http://amzn.to/1xt93sY

Check Out My Other Books

Below you'll find some of my other books also available on Amazon and Kindle. Search for these titles on the Amazon website to find them.

Paleo Free Diet Guide for Beginners: Over 50 Paleo Free Recipes for Optimal Health & Fast Weight Loss

Paleo Desserts: Satisfy Your Sweet Tooth With Over 100 Quick & Easy Paleo Dessert Recipes & Paleo Baking Recipes

Raw Food Diet Guide: Lose Weight Quickly, Achieve Optimal Health & Feel Energized with the Raw Food Diet & Raw Food Recipes

Clean Eating Guide: Lose Weight Quickly, Achieve Optimal Health & Feel Energized with Clean Eating For Busy Families & Clean Eating Recipes

Alkaline Diet Guide: Lose Weight Quickly, Achieve Optimal Health & Feel Energized with the Alkaline Diet & Alkaline Recipes

Coconut Flour Recipes for Optimal Health & Quick Weight Loss: Gluten Free Recipes for Celiac Disease, Gluten Sensitivities & Paleo Free Diets

Almond Flour Recipes for Optimal Health & Quick Weight Loss: Gluten Free Recipes for Celiac Disease, Gluten Sensitivities & Paleo Free Diets

Wheat Free Diet for Beginners: Lose Weight Quickly, Achieve Optimal Health & Feel Energized with Gluten Free Recipes for Celiac Disease, Gluten Sensitivities & Paleo Free Diets

Detox Diet Guide: Lose Weight Quickly, Achieve Optimal Health & Feel Energized Through the 10 Day Detox

Sugar Detox Guide for Beginners: Lose Weight Quickly, Achieve Optimal Health, Feel Energized & Eliminate Sugar Cravings Naturally

Ketogenic Diet Guide for Beginners: How to Achieve Rapid Weight Loss, Optimal Health & Unstoppable Energy with Ketogenic Diet Recipes

Anti Inflammatory Diet for Beginners: Lose Weight Fast, Optimize Health, Slow Aging, Fight Inflammation, Conquer Pain & Increase Energy with the Anti Inflammation Diet Recipes

One Last Thing...

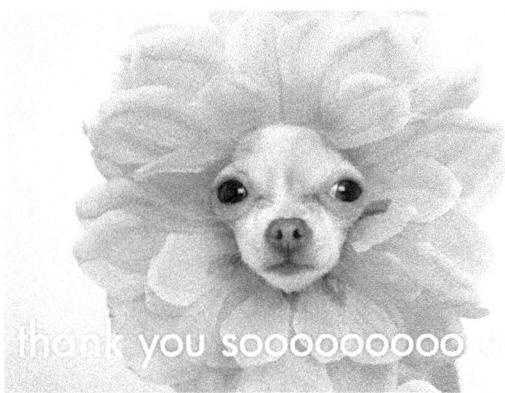

If you believe that this book is worth sharing, would you please take the time to let others know how it affected your life? If it turns out to make a difference in the lives of others, they will be forever grateful to you, as will I.

www.ingramcontent.com/pod-product-compliance
Lightning Source LLC
Chambersburg PA
CBHW070502290526
45790CB00003B/1059